50 Million Pounds In America

By Tara Christopher

PROLOGUE

Shallow (wo)men believe in luck. Strong (wo)men believe in cause and effect.
-Ralph Waldo Emerson

When people ask me why they *need* to change, I always answer, "Be Cause." Not one word. Two words.

Be. Cause.

It is not a mistake in printing. It is a call to action. What do I mean by BE CAUSE?

The Cause. You must find what drives you – your goals for yourself on a personal level and what you want your place in the world to be. You must find your mission, your CAUSE, and then you must…

Be it. It is quite simple conceptually, although too often it's difficult to achieve. Not knowing your CAUSE is probably at the heart of why you may have suffered disappointments in the past. You merely did things because you were expected to, or you were pressured into doing them, and you had not clearly identified your personal goals and what lasting effects you wanted for yourself and the world around you.

Be Cause means you must completely *be* your *cause* and once you achieve that state you will find there is absolutely nothing you cannot accomplish.

In this book and in the accompanying videos associated with each chapter –available absolutely free to buyers of this book – I will teach you how to find a cause that will inspire you. I will also show you things you can do to immerse yourself in your cause so that action, and change, become second nature to you.

The central part of Be Cause is about body and spirit: a technique I call *The Granite Method*. Your body and mind <u>must</u> be in prime working order to pursue and achieve your cause. *The Granite Method* and I will get you there.

A key part of *The Granite Method* is learning how to detoxify your mind and body of all the negative influences – chemical, philosophical, emotional – using a methodology I've nicknamed *Tara-fying*.

Fear not, *The Granite Method* and *Tara-fying* are not hocus-pocus and they will never put you at risk physically, emotionally, or financially. That's just not what I'm about. I've written this book because I've witnessed so many of my clients achieve things with their bodies and in their personal and professional lives that they never thought possible. Many of them have urged me to share it with you. So, here I am! What I'll be telling you about is largely brand new research concerning ways to get and stay mentally and physically fit, partly common sense, with a sprinkling of my own client-proven techniques for reaching new heights.

Come with me on this journey, and stick with me. Your cause awaits!

CHAPTER ONE

***The Yesterday's the past, tomorrow's the future, but
today is a gift.
That's why it's called the present.***
-Bil Keane, Cartoonist

"There Is No Tomorrow!" The fictional character, Apollo
Creed, yells at Rocky Balboa in the movie, *Rocky III*,
when Rocky is not giving his all during training.
Demoralized from an earlier shellacking at the powerful
hands of Clubber Lang and despondent after the death of
his long time trainer, Mickey, who was like a father to
him, Rocky refuses to put up a fight in the ring against
Apollo as he's preparing Rocky for a rematch against
Lang.

"Damn, Rock, Come on! What's the matter with you?"
Apollo questions.

Rocky responds, "Tomorrow. Let's do it tomorrow."

"There is no tomorrow," Apollo screams. "THERE IS
NO TOMORROW! THERE IS NO TOMORROW!"

Rocky's attitude is familiar in real life. We know we have
to make changes in order to be happy, to be fit, to be
healthy, to be successful, and yet we push change off to
tomorrow. We delay even thinking about why we should
change and what specifically we should be doing,
believing that *tomorrow* will be different – that somehow
tomorrow will magically bring us the time and insight

and inspiration we need to improve our lives. Tomorrow hardly ever delivers, however, and by relegating change to tomorrow, we allow ourselves to descend farther into unhappiness and ill health since our bodies and minds are always in motion – never still and always going either forward, or sinking backward. By saying you will do something tomorrow, you risk digging an even deeper hole for your body and spirit. So Apollo Creed was giving Rocky invaluable advice – that there is only today.

If the fictional Rocky had waited for *tomorrow* who knows what could have happened? He could have sunk deeper into despair and decided he wasn't ready to take on Lang. Or that missing day's worth of training could have made all the difference in the fight, propelling Rocky to a cataclysmic loss and prematurely to that half-satisfying career as a restaurant owner. Or perhaps Adrian would have left a pessimistic and paunchy Rocky because he was just not the man she married. If Rocky had waited until *tomorrow*, maybe there wouldn't have been Rocky IV, V, VI, and VII, denying audiences all that entertainment and satisfaction (excluding Rocky V which, critics agreed, was a stinker).

"The best preparation for tomorrow is doing your best today."
–H. Jackson Brown, Inspirational Author

The lesson we should take from the Rocky example is that change begins now. That tomorrow is merely to *build on* the progress we have propelled into it from today. There really is no tomorrow unless we start now.

Trust me, in the scheme of things, it all makes sense. *Tomorrow* is merely an excuse, an illusion. All we really have is <u>today</u>.

And while tomorrow is an illusion, *yesterday* is an obstacle. It hinders progress because you're either resting on laurels or kicking yourself for mistakes made. Do not, do not, do not criticize for having gained weight – or eating an entire box of donuts. DO NOT blame yourself for having squandered thousands of dollars on get-rich-quick schemes. And please do not criticize yourself for having done nothing yesterday. It's a trap that prevents you from movie forward. It's an excuse that leads to unfair labels about you:

"I'm just lazy."

"I don't have self control."

"I'm meant to be a failure."

Do NOT carry the incredible burden of guilt from yesterday. Only remember the lessons!

This book is here to help you answer the first questions – your *cause* – and since we have already answered the *when* (TODAY!), we will also help you answer the HOW. Fortunately, the *how* does not involve having to swallow raw eggs or do one-handed push-ups. It is, you'll be happy to know, much simpler. All you need is to do first is to look inside yourself to answer truthfully what you really want from life. To have more energy? To look better in a bathing suit? To be able to dress for success? To feel happier? To actually *feel* healthy deep inside, from your bones to your brain? To be able to go toe-to-toe with your own metaphorical Clubber Lang? (The quiz in the next chapter will help you identify your Cause.

What is the cause that will drive you to make big changes in your life? And what simple things can you start doing TODAY that will prepare you for tomorrow? This book will serve as your guide in three important areas – Mind, Fitness, Nutrition. I've found that all three areas are interrelated. When you make progress in one area, it can nurture success in the others, with a little guidance and a healthy amount of persistence. And when you conquer all three aspects of your inner life, you become the person people are attracted to since you will truly have it all together, in one fulfilled package.

In those specific sections about Mind, Fitness, and Nutrition and in the accompanying videos, I'll also describe the ways in which we overtly, and without knowing, undercut our minds and bodies by polluting the fragile systems that are supposed to be protecting us. I'll describe *Tara-fying* and the simple things I recommend to ensure your body is working at peak performance and is as impervious to harmful forces from the outside.

First let me give you an example of a client of mine.

A few years ago a thirty-five year old woman named Candice came to me seeking help because she wanted to get in better health prior to a scheduled stomach bypass operation. Her blood pressure was 190 over 95 and she was two-hundred-seventy pounds overweight. She had not yet materialized Type 2 Diabetes, but her doctor had told her that she was certainly on the fast path to a diabetes diagnosis, and she needed to lose weight and get her blood pressure into a more normal range. Weight loss medications had not worked for her and had actually aggravated her blood pressure condition, so the doctor pointedly described her rock-and-a hard-place situation: he could not perform the surgery on her and help her artificially reach a "healthier" state until she got herself in better shape so he could operate.

"It's ridiculous, isn't it?" Candice admitted. "I'm scared of the surgery and if I don't get my blood pressure under control, I could die on the table. And if I don't get thinner, I could die in my sleep."

It's not my job to diagnose people or recommend anything that would contradict doctor's orders, but when I studied Candice's sincere blue eyes and noticed her almost super-model'esque features, I suspected there was a more practical solution for her, that she could emerge safely out of the hole she allowed herself to sink into, and be transformed into a healthy, gorgeous, happier woman with most of her life ahead of her. When I asked her why she was choosing surgery instead of simpler solutions – the "stick-and-move," (to borrow a boxing phrase) of a smart regimen of diet, exercise, and balanced nutrition – she told me she wanted something fast and relatively easy. But her eyes burned with determination, a quality I knew she could turn into an asset as she tackled a more reasonable solution that she could follow for the rest of her life.

"I have to do this, Tara," she said, as if to convince herself as much as me. "I've done everything."

"Really? Everything?" I answered.

"Yeah, acupuncture, the cabbage soup diet, the cookie diet, the grapefruit diet, hypnosis, South Beach," she listed in alphabetical order. "Everything."

"Let me guess," I shot back. "Acupuncture and hypnosis worked for a few days until the placebo effect wore off. And you'd actually lose some weight with the crazy diets until your body was so full of poison you'd get headaches or throw up. Or give up."

She nodded shamefully.

The Placebo Effect is worth talking about here. In science and pseudo-science, researchers and marketers have found that in studies in which subjects or consumers are given a placebo – an ineffectual drug or product (a "sugar pill") – twenty to thirty percent of people report "positive effects" from having used the placebo, even though there is no scientific reason for it. What I like to highlight about The Placebo Effect is that it is powerful proof about **the power of the mind.** If you truly believe something will work for you, and you have tools to turn that belief into positive,

CONSISTENT action, eventually the effect becomes real and permanent.

After a number of delicate questions, I learned that someone Candice worked with had somewhat callously recommended surgery to her and then when she saw a well-produced and supremely convincing commercial on television for gastric bypass, she concluded "it was destiny." Candice called the toll-free number for the clinic advertising its services, and fancying herself a doer and wanting so terribly to wear regular-sized clothes and start looking beautiful to *someone,* she decided then and there that she would do it, with surprisingly little research.

When the timing was right – when her eyes searched my face for some alternative - I laid on her my signature line, "There is no magic cure. No one-step, be-beautiful-overnight solution. No one has invented one that won't increase your chances of dying tragically. It's the disappointing truth. BUT… there is a solution and it's not a fad diet or a pill or surgery, it's what I call The Granite Method."

"The Granite Method. What is that?"

"Imagine that you are a large block of raw granite. And you have four tools. A large and heavy mallet. A carving tool sharp enough to cut through rough stone. And a polishing tool."

"What do you use them for?" Candice asked.

"The Mallet represents exercise. It's hard work. You slam it against the stone to chip away at it, slowly but methodically. You push yourself but you only do as much as you absolutely can. You chip away at the granite a bit at a time. A little bit each day. But you have to do it every day. I'll be here to encourage you.'

"What's the carving tool for?" She continued.

"The carving tool represents nutrition, " I told her. "And something I call *Tara-fying*. Your body must be in balance and we have to get you there sensibly. No cabbage soup or cookie overload and no starvation. Small, smart changes, making sure that you're getting all the nutrients and vitamins you need, through food, water, and supplements if you absolutely need them. It's as much about detoxifying as it is about nutrifying. Simple techniques I'll teach you that have been the keys to success for so many people."

I gave Candice many notable examples of famous people who had found regimens that were keeping their bodies and minds operating optimally. Famous comedian and television actor Dick Van Dyke has been an icon of health, energy, and vitality ever since his days as the star of a television series, *The Dick Van Dyke Show*, in the early 1960's. Now ninety years old (as of this writing), Dick Van Dyke has a simple formula for health – a positive attitude, a joy of life, a "constant state of motion," and sensible eating. Not at all a stickler for dieting, Dick allows himself ice cream every day but in moderation… and dancing with his young wife every day. Dick has had his demons, as many of us have had; he spent many of his young years a victim of alcohol abuse, but he learned the technique of using small steps to achieve radical change at Alcoholics Anonymous. That methodology of gradual, persistent change is a central philosophy of this book – meaningful change comes from chipping away at a problem, not searching for quick-fixes. There are other techniques that will be helpful in your quest for change, and I'll be showing you those too.

"Let me guess," Candice offered, "The polishing tool represents the mind?"

"Very good," I answered. "It all comes together with the right attitude about the rattling noise that change makes in your body. The grumbles in your stomach on occasion, the creaking of your joints and your muscles, and the doubts bouncing around in your head. But if you hang in there for enough time, and you stay confident and persistent and *positive* (like our friend Dick Van Dyke), you will notice obvious changes in how you look and how you feel, and how you view the world. It really is miraculous."

"You said there were four tools. What's the fourth tool?" Candice asked.

"A pencil," I said like I was delivering a punch-line. "You use it first. To design the changes you want to make, and draw what you'll look like when the initial work is done. And you use the pencil to rewrite your story, because you've been living an incomplete and one that does not represent who you are or what you want to be."

"So where do I begin?"

"It starts with the hunt for your CAUSE."

CHAPTER TWO

The Cause Test is your first step to the new and improved you. After all, how can you embark on an adventure unless you know the reason you're going? This test will let you assess the areas of your life in which you're not maximizing your well-being.

The score at the end of this first quiz within the test – which has been culled from the work of Rochelle Forrest, a leading expert in the field of health and fitness – will point out trouble areas. The result of the first set of questions will then lead you to subsequent quizzes in later sections of this chapter that will allow us to drill down further.

I'll then help you make sense of it all in Chapter 3 and come up with your CAUSE.

[In this section, give yourself 1 point for every Yes answer, subtract 1 point for every No answer.]

Physical Health and Nutrition

1. I tend to fall asleep easily most of the time.

Yes/Agree. No/Disagree _____

2. Do you ever think before eating, *"Is this a wise investment for my body?"*

Yes/Agree. No/Disagree _____

3. I wake up full of energy in the morning.

 Yes/Agree. No/Disagree_____

4. I can walk for more than 10 minutes without getting out of breath.

Yes/Agree. No/Disagree_____

5. The quality of the food I eat is important to me.

Yes/Agree. No/Disagree_____

6. I *infrequently* eat fast food or deep fried foods.

Yes/Agree. No/Disagree_____

7. I stay aware of news about supplements and vitamins and of their benefits and drawbacks.

Yes/Agree. No/Disagree_____

8. I work out at least three times a week for 30 minutes.

Yes/Agree. No/Disagree_____

9. I do <u>not</u> have chronic or recurrent pain (back pain, migraines, etc.)

Yes/Agree. No/Disagree_____

10. I am at my ideal weight.

Yes/Agree. No/Disagree_____

11. When I go to the pool or the beach, I am never self-conscious.

Yes/Agree. No/Disagree_____

12. When I look in the mirror, I do not see ANY areas that I would like to change.

Yes/Agree. No/Disagree_____

13. I am confident I am doing everything I can to protect my health.

Yes/Agree. No/Disagree_____

Section Total _____

Emotional Health and Well-being

1. I communicate my feelings and my needs easily, calmly and with confidence.

Yes/Agree. No/Disagree_____

2. I do NOT hold grudges nor find it difficult to forgive others and myself.

Yes/Agree. No/Disagree_____

3. I am confident in my skills and abilities.

Yes/Agree. No/Disagree_____

4. I do NOT have a temper and am always in control of my emotions.

Yes/Agree. No/Disagree_____

5. I enjoy close relationships with friends and loved ones.

Yes/Agree. No/Disagree_____

6. In reviewing my life so far, I do NOT wish I had accomplished more.

Yes/Agree. No/Disagree_____

7. I would describe myself as happy most of the time.

Yes/Agree No/Disagree_____

8. I do NOT carry the weight of painful past events in my heart.

Yes/Agree. No/Disagree_____

Section Total _____

Mental Health and Clear Thinking

1. I choose positive thoughts even in difficult situations.

Yes/Agree. No/Disagree_____

2. I rarely find it difficult to motivate myself.

Yes/Agree. No/Disagree_____

3. I keep an open mind and look out for new ideas and opportunities.

Yes/Agree. No/Disagree_____

4. I tend to expect the best and rarely worry about outcomes.

Yes/Agree. No/Disagree_____

5. I feel like I can accomplish anything if I set my mind to it.

Yes/Agree. No/Disagree_____

6. My mind hardly ever runs negative tapes and if it does, I can easily stop them.

Yes/Agree. No/Disagree_____

7. I do my best in every situation and give a 100%.

Yes/Agree. No/Disagree_____

8. I never make excuses for myself.

Yes/Agree. No/Disagree_____

Section Total _____

If you scored between 11 and 13 in the Physical Health and Nutrition section of the quiz, congratulations, you're rare and you can skip to the Goals Intensive toward the end of this chapter. But if you're like most of us, you scored 10 or below in the Physical Health and Nutrition section, which means we should drill down further in the Physical Health Intensive below to find out if your WHY is more about fitness or nutrition or a combination of both.

If you did not get a <u>perfect</u> score in the Mental Health and Emotional Health sections (8 out of 8 in both), it's possible you're blocking yourself from making progress with regards to your physical health. In order for you to be successful with the Granite Method, you MUST be positive and optimistic always, even if you don't think it's in your "nature."

Everyone therefore should take the last quiz in this chapter. (The Goals Intensive) since it will tell us more about what will motivate you to make improvements in your health and well-being.

(The following health quiz is a compilation of research conducted by the Michigan Department of Health & Human Services, the education services of the Office of the Surgeon General of the United States, and Health.Gov.)

PHYSICAL HEALTH INTENSIVE

Cigarette Smoking & Alcohol/Drug Use

Always_____ Sometimes_____ Never_____

If you are currently a non-smoker and non-drug user, give yourself 20 points.

- I smoke, but do so rarely and only for stress-relief._____ (2 points)
- I smoke but under 1 pack per day._____ (-5 points)

- I smoke more than 1 pack per day._____(-20 points)
- I am a casual drinker, no more than 2-3 drinks per week._____(5 points)
- I drink every day/ night._____(-5 points)
- I have a been known to "black out" when I drink socially._____(-20 points)
- I must have alcohol to feel comfortable in social settings._____(-5 points)
- I must have prescription drugs or illegal drugs to have a good time in social settings._____(-10 points)
- I rely on prescription or illegal drugs to deal with my stresses._____ (-15 points)
- I have had serious problems when I'm under the influence of drugs or alcohol. (DWI arrest, loud or violent arguments, disturbing the peace, car accidents, etc.)_____(-30 points)

Smoking/Alcohol/Drug Use Score:_____

Any negative number in this section should serve as a warning for you to seek outside help for smoking cessation and / or alcohol and drug rehabilitation. While the fitness and nutrition help this book provides will be useful for everyone, this should <u>not</u> be your first stop on your road to better health. If you scored in the negative numbers in this section, please seek outside help immediately.

Physical Activity and Exercise

1. I accumulate 30 or more minutes of moderate physical activity at least 5 days a week (e.g.. walking, yard work, golf w/o a power cart . . .) or engage in vigorous exercise for 20 minutes at least 3 times a week (e.g. running, swimming, aerobics, etc.)

5 (always)   2 (sometimes)   0 (never)
_____(your score)

2. I do things like taking stairs instead of elevators and don't worry about getting the closest available parking spot.

2 (always)   1 (sometimes)   0 (never)
_____(your score)

3. I do exercises that enhance my muscle tone and flexibility at least 2 - 3 times per week.

3 (always)   1 (sometimes)   0 (never)
_____(your score)

4. I enjoy a variety of recreational activities with friends and family.

2 (always)   1 (sometimes)   0 (never)
_____(your score)

5. I engage in regular (daily, weekly) organized sports such as tennis, racket ball, basketball, speed biking, etc.)

5 (always)   2 (sometimes)   0 (never)
_____(your score)

6. I engage in low-impact pastimes such as bowling, leisure biking, short-distance hiking, etc. at least once per month.

2 (always)   1 (sometimes)   0 (never)
_____(your score)

7. I receive professional massages (Swedish, Thai, deep tissue, etc.) at least once per month.

2 (always)   1 (sometimes)   0 (never)
_____(your score)

8. I would describe my sex life as active, loving, and as frequent as desired.

4 (always)   2 (sometimes)   0 (never)
_____(your score)

Physical Activity and Exercise Score:_____

If you scored between 21 and 25 in this section, BRAVO! You are living in the perfect range. You're active and participating in life and your body is a well-oiled machine; you are maximizing your chances of living a long, illness-free life!

If you scored between 10 and 19 in this section, you have areas of improvement and you should focus on the physical fitness sections of this book and all of the support materials (videos and newsletters). Fear not, though, getting to the 21 to 25 range will be very straightforward for you. It's a matter of making relatively small changes that will add up to big gains.

If you scored under 10 in this section, don't be disheartened! Your motto from here on out should be GET MOVING! Start with the small changes – taking the stairs instead of the elevator and making sure you walk instead of drive - and start treating yourself to things like bowling outings with friends and monthly massages. And begin by monitoring your movements with Step Counting apps on your phone or in a wristband. Start with a daily target of 5000 steps with the goal being to get to 10,000 steps every day, rain or shine.

>See later sections for more advice on staying active and getting fit.

So we've briefly covered physical activity and we've started to identify how and where you can make improvements. Now it's time for you to dig deep and ask yourself what will *really* motivate you.

The GOALS INTENSIVE

For each question, take a moment to think before you commit your answer to the pages. These answers will help you come up with the images you will play over and over in your head as you work hard to make changes in your life.

Get out a #2 pencil or, if you're brave, a pen, and write down your answers within this book. This will serve as your vision book for what you want to achieve from the Granite Method.

- Imagine it's two years from now and someone has asked you to pose for a picture in front of a beautiful landscape. What do you look like? How much better do you look then as compared to now? (Remember, this is not at all based on your current reality, this needs to be real in your brain. **You need to really believe that what you see is what you ARE.)**

- Imagine it's two years from now and you're comfortable in a bathing suit. Are you comfortable in your own skin? What will it take to get you there?

- Imagine it's two years from now and someone asks you to join them for a long hike through a beautiful mountain side, how do you feel? Are you confident you're up to the physical challenge?

- In two years, how will you describe yourself? (Confident? Financially secure? Physically fit?

- It's the present. What short-term goals would you like to achieve? (Is it to be able to fit into a slim gown for an upcoming wedding or to fit into a pair of jeans that you used to be able to slip into or do you just want to feel stronger and healthier – like you once did?) Remember, it's short term. You will need to think of a series of small steps to get you there, and you should keep in mind that you'll be living "one day at a time."

- What other goals would you like to achieve? (Climb the peaks of a nearby mountain range? Go on a ten-mile hike? Be the leader of your own company? Be a great role model for your children?)

*

Congratulations! You're on the path to a better, healthier, happier you!

In the coming chapters, we'll follow Candice through her adventure and we'll meet other people with different focus areas, whether they're within fitness, nutrition, or their mental commitment.

In the next chapter, I'll tell you how you can take what you've learned within this chapter and apply it to a sensible, effective, AND FUN plan! So, keep reading!

CHAPTER THREE

"Knowing is not enough, we must APPLY.
Willing is not enough, we must DO."
-Bruce Lee, Martial Arts Icon

So by now you should do by now you should have uncovered some possibilities for your *CAUSE*. Why are you embarking on a mission to feel better, look better, be better? You should have been able to identify short term goals - like, wanting to fit into jeans that you once could fit into, or, not being ashamed to take off your T-shirt at the beach, or, being able to climb a set of stairs without getting winded.

You should have also started identifying long-term goals for yourself. Do you want to live long past retirement age? Do you want to be able to stop taking certain kinds of medications that you now rely on? (Lipitor? Nexium? Valium?) Or perhaps you want to:

- Start a business
- Write a book
- Create a piece of art
- Become a public speaker
- Start a foundation

I have to emphasize the importance of your Cause again. Your Cause is your fire. You don't have to be reminded of it. It's just there. You don't have ask yourself *why* you need to pursue it, you'll always be asking *how* to achieve it, even when the inevitable disappointments happen or obstacles block your path.

It's simple. By defining your short term and long-term missions, YOUR CAUSE, you will have the power to push through the difficult parts to achieve your goals.

When we have something negative or tragic happen in our lives, the first question we ask is why. This should also be our first question when we are about to do something positive. By knowing your cause in life, we can nurture the positive aspects of the changes we are making and the lessons we are learning, even when setbacks happen.

And yes, there will be setbacks.

They come from the outside or from within. So the question you must ask yourself before you start is: "Is my cause bigger than any, and all, negative forces? And if it's not, how do I find the strength to still take action?"

When Candice, my client who came to me before a scheduled stomach bypass operation, was sorting through her reasons for the surgery and for the alternatives I was hoping she would pick instead, she easily came up with the obvious reasons:

- To look better than she had ever looked;
- To lose at least one hundred pounds;

- To get to a level of comfort with how she looked to start dating for the first time in her life;
- To feel worthy of being loved;

And the big one…

- To make radical changes she was never courageous enough to attempt.

Candice had hit on the largest negative force that threatens to thwart the search for a cause:

FEAR.

This is a negative force that comes from within. In most cases, the fear is unfounded and it can be subconscious. Many successful people and countless great writers have written about fear, since it is such a common obstacle to great success. As Henry Ford said:

"One of the greatest discoveries a (wo)man makes, one of her/his great surprises, is to find (s)he can do what (s)he was afraid (s)he couldn't do."

The best way to fight fear is to attack that enemy head on. Action defeats fear, especially if the action itself is what you fear most. So you want to be a speaker, but you fear being laughed at or booed. The best way to defeat that fear is to schedule a speaking engagement and follow the advice of the tennis shoe manufacturer,

Nike… *Just Do It!* What is the worst thing that could happen? You'll be publicly embarrassed. Perhaps you won't be invited to speak in front of those people again. So what? You should coach yourself to turn that grand disappointment into a lesson on how to do it better the next time!

You have an offer to get involved in a network marketing business at a low cost. You love the idea, but you have this deep-seeded fear of failing. Guess what? You just might fail, but why fear that? If you do not try, you have no chance of failing, but you also have no chance of success. Fear is your enemy, so treat it as such. Do we allow enemies into our home? Do we allow enemies into our business?

A client of mine, Sam from Nevada, called me because he was crippled by fear. His Cause was that he wanted to make more money for his growing family and to pay for a new house he had bought near Las Vegas. Sam had quit his job as a blackjack dealer, having grown tired of life working in a casino, and the constant "clank, clank, clank" of the environment.

"It damned on me one day that it was a dead-end," Sam told me. "The most I would ever make at that job was written in stone."

Sam had left to help a friend start a technology company selling innovative software to handle conference calls for big multinational companies. Problem was, Sam found that he was scared about making cold calls. Not an uncommon affliction of people in sales and in any multilevel marketing enterprise. But Sam's success was directly related to his ability to call hundreds of people in one day, in the hopes he could get one or two people a day (qualified leads) whose names he could pass on to a salesperson in the field.

"I can't do it, Tara," Sam moaned. "It's like my cell phone weighs a hundred pounds."

After a series of questions, it became clear to me that Sam's problem was fear. Fear of rejection superficially. Fear of failure deep inside of him. Plus a healthy amount of laziness. But the fear was blocking his success. And the laziness was preventing him from knocking down the fear.

"First, Sam," I told him. "The laziness is common. But you know, there's only one thing laziness leads to. It's DEATH. People spend their lives sleeping or watching TV or drinking or drugging. It's lazy. Laziness leads to death. Remember that."

"Okay, but why am I afraid?"

"Forget the reasons WHY, Sam," I urged. "Focus on the *how*. And in your case, the how is action. Just pick up the phone, read the script and enjoy both the rejections and the moment you first get a sense that someone is interested in what you're saying. And when you hear it, think to yourself that there's money it in for you."

"*Thinking will not overcome fear but action will.*"
–W. Clement Stone, Self-Help Book Author

In many cases, it is our family and friends who can sway our thought processes into an "I can't" attitude. "You didn't go to school for that…" or "Your uncle Frank tried that and lost his shirt!" The comments and attitudes of our friends and family can be an enemy from the outside. These people are committing that dream killing initiative, but you still have a choice. Will you accept defeat before you even started? Even though this enemy is attacking from the outside, the true enemy that needs to be defeated is on the inside. It all goes back to fear and insecurity. Of course, you love and respect the people who are trying to kill your dream, but you must realize they do not live your life. They do not know what you know and they will not have to suffer the consequences. So why allow them to kill your search for a Cause? You have to just keep moving because you are worth it.

Another client of mine, Jim, had this dream of starting his own bakery. Heather, Jim's wife, always loved the many pastries and pies Jim made during his off hours from the factory job he had worked for 14 years. Jim and Heather talked about the bakery idea often and they carefully considered why he should start a bakery. There were several key *whys*:

- Jim was skilled at baking;

- They were empty-nesters, as their two children were in college;
- Jim and Heather had $120,000 saved, so they believed that they could survive through the start-up;
- Jim had shared his baked goods with fellow employees, friends, family, and neighbors and they unanimously agreed he had the right stuff to start his own bakery;
- Jim's best friend was an executive at a major bank, and he told Jim he was willing to help him get financing.

All of these whys gave Jim and Heather the inspiration. But then Jim was unexpectedly laid off while he was looking for a location and obtaining financing for his bakery business. The factory where he had worked for many years had to cut back, and Jim was on the list to receive a pink slip.

Fear took hold and Jim was ready to scuttle plans to start his own business. Heather sat him down after having read an early article that would become the core of *The Granite Method* and would lead me to write *Be Cause*.

"Jim, we found our Cause, we should start a bakery, so you can't quit now," Heather urged. "If you try to turn this setback into a positive, you'll find that it's easy. You don't have a job now holding you back. You can focus on getting the perfect bakery set up. We have savings and Brian is obtaining the financing. We have the Cause answered, so let's start a bakery."

Heather was right! Jim's fear disappeared.

They ended up starting their business, working out of their home to grow a catering business first. Within eight months, Heather and Jim had collected enough successful stories and a network of potential clients for their store, and one year later they opened J&H Fineries at the exact location Jim had dreamed of being where a store of his own would open.

Now J&H has a robust catering business that supplements a healthy walk-in and holiday enterprise. Jim and Heather recently quadrupled their business almost overnight by starting an online operation and selling and shipping baked goods across the country. Jim has found that he is skilled at managing his business while Heather has demonstrated a skill at marketing, managing employees, and charming customers.

Jim overcame his fear of failure and has found incredible success in the process. Only action overcomes fear. Jim and Heather have proved it definitively.

*

So this is your place to list your possible Causes. And list your fears too. Remember, the one rule is that your Cause has to be strong enough to overcome the fears. And then when you've stared at your lists long enough – hours, not days – **TAKE ACTION.**

You are the master of your destiny. When others are standing still, you just need to keep moving, because you have determined your Cause, and when you move on with your goals, your family and friends will take notice. **You will BE your Cause!** Some will continue to complain, or tell you stories of grand failures. Many of them might be trying to "protect you," others might be jealous because they have not found ways to overcome their own fears. Bottom line is that you should NOT LISTEN. Please remember…

> *"There is no tomorrow!"*
> Apollo Creed, Fictional Boxer

Fear can be a sly enemy. You must always be on guard against this foe. One of the primary defenses against fear is to stay clear of negative thoughts and people. While this is not always possible, you must make a decision daily to not allow fear to have any place in your life. When a negative thought attempts to enter, it should you to take action. Fill your mind with positive thoughts. Imagine a ticking clock. If you wallow in the negatives, your odds of quitting and pushing change off until tomorrow will grow substantially.

The secret to negative thoughts is that they are even more of an illusion than *tomorrow*. Unless your problem is bio-chemical – and so few of them really are – your negative thoughts merely require that you shift your focus to something positive.

- Drive to a scenic overlook and marvel at the beauty,
- Read your favorite book
- Watch an inspiring YouTube video,
- Watch one of my inspirational videos,
- Focus on something good in your life,
- Think of how making progress will make you feel,
- Trust that things will be "better in the morning" (they often are!),
- DECIDE to feel positive,
- Talk to the most positive, optimistic, friendly person you know.
- Make sure to identify the negative thoughts as you have them so you have change the conditions that may have led you to feel them.

Any of these activities, inspire your brain to produce feel-good endorphins, which will vanquish the negatives and will train your brain to act differently.

The other thing you should do is stop being anywhere near nay-sayers, malcontents, and buzz-killers. We all know them – people who love being downers. Stay away from them AT ALL COSTS.

CHAPTER FOUR

*"We do not stop exercising because we grow old –
we grow old because we stop exercising."*
-Dr. Kenneth Cooper, first advocate of the benefits of
"Aerobics"

The Granite Method STEP ONE

Break out your heavy mallet to start chipping away at
the raw granite block that you are!

Our minds and bodies need constant exercise. Does this
mean you should go out and purchase a gym
membership? If that will give you the inspiration to
exercise, maybe it would be a good thing, but a person
does not need a gym to exercise.

In fact, I have found that a gym membership for many
people is absolutely NOT the right approach. If you're
not already in good shape, a gym environment - with all
the preening and propositioning that goes on all around –
can be disheartening! Some gyms are as much a
showcase for fit bodies than a place to get one.

"I went to one of those luxury gyms, Tara. It had a juice
bar and a sauna and a store with clothes that would never
fit me even if I lost a hundred pounds!" Candice
admitted to me, almost in tears. "And I could see people
talking about me when they spotted me huffing and
puffing on the treadmill. One guy, who was a little bit
too muscle-bound to look like he was smart, actually

came up to me to see if I needed water or help changing the speed."

"Maybe he liked you," I consoled.

"Doubt it," Candice joked. "He probably didn't want to have to perform CPR on me."

Just because one person goes to a gym, or runs, or swims for their exercise routine does not mean you have to follow their lead. Just because everyone is *spinning* does not mean you have to buy all the latest bike fashions.

Exercise does not have to be toil. Maybe walking or hiking is fun for you... that is, most definitely, exercise. How about ice or roller-skating? Both of those sports can be great for the body. There are a lot of physical things a person can do to get exercise.

Consider:

- Yoga
- Bike riding
- Swimming
- Tennis
- Ballroom Dancing
- Aquaerobics
- Circuit Training
- Boxing
- Self-Defense Classes

The common goal is for you to get out and use your

body in physical ways.

Candice, in her quest to get into shape to be ready for gastric bypass surgery, started walking into her town to get groceries, instead of driving, When she managed that comfortably, she then would walk everywhere she could, even planning hikes by herself on weekends with no goals attached, except to *be with the woods.*

There are some individuals who have a difficult time getting out of their house or apartment. There are still many ways to exercise in the comfort of your home. You don't need a gym, or a lot of expensive exercise equipment.

Here are a few ideas of exercises you can do at home. We all know these, or have heard of them, but it's a good way to access your level of fitness and start being proactive:

- **Push-ups:** You can start with your knees on the floor, or do a full push-up with your toes. Just spread your arms shoulder width, and push your upper body up. Lower and repeat. Set a goal of fives. Do five at first. Push yourself! And when five are easy, add five and do ten push-ups. Keep going with that formula up until 20. Then keep adding five until fifty. And so on. Yes, it's tough but, trust me, you will start to see amazing changes in your upper body, and your strength, once you're doing twenty push-ups with relative ease.

- **Crunches:** For your abdomen, you simply lay on your back with your knees up. With your hands behind your head, lift your upper body toward your knees. Lower and repeat. Do not force your head up with your hands, though, (it's not an arm exercise!), make sure to lift your upper body with abdominal muscles. Try sets of ten, and like above, add ten when the first ten starts to get easy to do. When you can do fifty easily, you are in amazing shape!
- **Squats:** With your hands above your head, lower your upper body using your knees to flex. Raise and repeat. For this exercise, push yourself PAST when your thighs BURN. Vary this exercise by pausing in the down position. Also, start with doing squats for thirty seconds, then add thirty seconds each time you think it's getting too easy. (Motivation: this exercise is great for your butt and thighs!)
- **Lunge:** Standing straight with your legs together, take one leg forward keeping your upper body straight. The leg that moves forward should have a bent knee forming a square pattern. Raise and repeat switching legs.
- **Side Lunge:** The same as the regular lunge, but to the side.   One Leg: Stand on one leg to the count of ten. Repeat using the other leg.
- **Hip Raises:** Lay flat on your back, and raise your hips holding to a count of five to ten. Lower and repeat.

These are just a sample of the many exercises you can do in the privacy of your home. It is recommended that before performing exercises, you should do stretches to free up your muscles so you do not harm them. Just do movements such as twirling your arms, legs and neck. Bend over and touch your toes. Do sideways bends. All of these will help you stretch your muscles so they will work properly when exercising.

Exercise Your Mind

While we need physical exercise, some people forget that our brains are an active muscle too. We need to exercise our brains. If we are always performing the same functions, our brains can get lazy. There are many ways to exercise our mental functions:

- Read books
- Play strategy games (chess, monopoly, etc…)
- Do puzzles
- Learn something new
- Train yourself to use the opposite hand from your dominant one
- Do a routine task in a different way
- Drive to work, school, or the supermarket by a different route
- Avoid Speed Dial – use your memory to dial numbers
- Have complex conversations – about news, history or current events – with friends

Sometimes just trying something new that you have never done can be a great way to give your brain some exercise. Maybe you would want to write a book, draw a picture, or any number of other things that will force your brain to have to react to different circumstances.

Another great way to exercise your brain is to mentor others. Not only are you helping yourself, but you are also helping another person and interacting with them in a unique way.

Exercising is a fundamental aspect in keeping your body and mind in the condition it was originally meant to be in. All it takes is just to keep on moving and stay in shape physically and mentally.

Our capacities and mind function shrink with routine. So this is as critical as physical activity.

CHAPTER FIVE

"A healthy body is a guest-chamber for the soul; a sick body is a prison."
–Sir Francis Bacon

The Granite Method– STEP TWO

Time to break out your carving tool. In this section we will talk about the need to deploy your carving tool while you're slugging way at your granite slab with the mallet also known as exercise. The two tools work in concert – one is not as effective without the other. The two together, though, can work miracles!

Our bodies are machinery that can endure multiple outside stresses, if we keep them perfectly tooled. With any machinery there is maintenance and upkeep that must be performed regularly. If we look at any type of machine, it cannot run non-stop without stopping for rest and maintenance, and it simply cannot function for long without the proper oils and fuels.

So why would our bodies be any different?

There are those certain laws of the body that are a given: if we get cut, we bleed. If we breathe in pollution, we cough and sneeze and contract illness. But, there are other laws of the body that are not quite as obvious, and we sometimes take these laws for granted. The laws that immediately come to mind are:

- We must tone and boost our bodies with the correct amount of exercise.
- We must allow our bodies to have sufficient sleep and rest.
- We must make sure our bodies get the proper amount of essential vitamins and minerals.
- We must protect our bodies from outside pollutants and harm, such as too much sun or other natural and man-made substances that can harm us overtly and covertly.

With so much conflicting research about nutrition, however, how do we sort through it all to find the essential truths? For example, Vitamin D has come into focus because of its strong connection to diseases like Multiple Sclerosis and Cancer – the lack of it in colder regions of the world because of less sun exposure seems to be connected to MS and the increased presence of Vitamin D due to healthy eating, sun exposure, and effective supplement use has been linked to decreased cancer rates.

"Vitamin D is most known for its beneficial effects on the skeleton, but, to me, its effects on cancer are much more significant," says Bruce W. Hollis, Ph.D., professor of pediatrics at the Medical University of South Carolina in Charleston.

In a study of 47,800 men, scientists at the Harvard School of Public Health reported that 1,500 IU daily of vitamin D reduced the risk of cancers of the digestive system by 43 percent. Another study from the University of California at San Diego of 1,760 women suggests that 2,700 IU daily may reduce the risk of breast cancer by 50 percent.

However, sun exposure raises the risk of skin cancer.

How do you resolve the conflict, not only with Vitamin D but with so many other vitamins and minerals that protect us from disease and illness, but may be difficult to consume through diet and pose a risk of over-consumption through supplements?

Humans have longed hunted for the Fountain Of Youth. In searching for the fountain, we have put our bodies through stresses that have aged it even more. Our search has defaulted to looking for quick fixes and we've been susceptible to over-bloated claims. From my observations of my clients and from combing through population studies regarding nutrition, I would estimate that for approximately 85% of the nation's population taking care of the body is not a primary focus. This is why we have such a high rate of diseases that are due to not obeying the laws of the body. Diseases such as:

- Diabetes
- Thyroid problems
- Heart diseases
- Cancer

It is time that we looked to our ancestors. For thousands of years, humans ate substances such as fruits, vegetables, nuts, fish, and other lean meats. In the

1800's, health problems and short life expectancies (on average 35-40 years of age for a man) came from events such as being run over by a runaway horse or a buffalo stampede (it was a risky time!), poor sanitation, and diseases caused by bacterias and viruses that modern science have now eradicated or kept in check. Today our life expectancies are much longer (74-79 years of age for a modern man) because of improved health care and sanitation, immunizations, access to clean, running water, and better nutrition.

However, recently researchers reported that for the first time life expectancies have been decreasing. People are not living as long as they did just a few years ago! The chief reason according to the researchers?

Obesity.

What would happen with the human population if the majority of us started obeying the laws of the body with respect to nutrition?

The fact is: if we all ingested food sources such as the nuts and seeds, veggies, fruits and fish, like early man did, we would be consuming daily nutrition loaded with the vitamins and minerals our bodies need. We still might take a supplement, for essential disease-fighting vitamins and minerals of which our bodies need a surplus (like Vitamin D) but we will be supplementing smartly and not haphazardly.

"But foods like salmon and green vegetables and some supplements are much more expensive than fast food!" Candice once yelled at me.

"It's an excuse, Candice," I interrupted. "You have to calculate the real cost! How much do you think diabetes will end up costing you? Not only in medical bills, but in lost productivity and decreased quality of life! What will that gastric bypass surgery cost? You can't tell me that if you had been eating right and exercising all along that you would still need to subject yourself to that cost and incredible risk. I can go on, Candice."

"Okay, go on," Candice teased.

"If you're just looking at the cost of the food," I answered. "Two dollars a day more than what you're spending now. But I actually think you're going to spend less. Being overweight and out of shape is much more expensive. You pick hiring an Uber or jumping in a cab instead of walking, even on nice days. You need expensive medications for things directly related to being overweight."

"Okay enough," Candice interrupted. "I get it."

"You have to live your Cause, Candice. You have to Be It and it will all suddenly seem so simple."

That was the turning point for Candice. Perhaps I had told her enough times and it had finally sunk in, or maybe she just wanted to stop hearing me say the same thing over and over again, but from that moment on, Candice got it. She knew that fixing her body and improving her life were merely a matter of BEING HER CAUSE. Candice wanted to feel whole and she yearned to be productive. She wanted to contribute to the world, and she wanted to love and be loved. That was her Cause and it only took that one last push for her to BE IT.

Soon after that confrontation over nutrition, Candice accepted what she needed to do. With me sitting next to her and holding her hand, Candice phoned her doctor and canceled her scheduled gastric bypass operation.

She says now she has never regretted having done it.

*

The Importance Of H2O

> *"Thousands have lived without love, not one without water."*
> W.H. Auden, Poet

Do you really understand the importance of H2O?

Water is not just an ordinary liquid, it is essential to life. Two-thirds of the adult body is made of it and every cell in the body needs it to keep working. Water regulates our body temperature through sweating and respiration, it lubricates our joints, it keeps our skin – the body's largest organ – moist and protective of the muscles underneath, and it flushes out toxins and waste through urination.

The longest a person can go without water is about one week, but that's generous. The average person can only live three or four days without water. The shortest is two or three hours in broiling heat.

Water is one of the primary elements on our planet. Without water, Earth would be a desert, incapable of sustaining indigenous life.

We must replenish our body's water supply by drinking and by eating the right foods. Most likely more than you currently drink. And we must drink it not only for survival; we rarely allow ourselves to become dangerously dehydrated. We must drink water because those cells that we mentioned need sufficient supplies to remove waste and toxins quickly and to convert the food we eat into basic nutrients and into energy. A body running below ideal levels of H_2O struggles to stay in balance and becomes much more susceptible to illness and more likely to react badly to physical and mental stresses.

So how much water should a person drink daily? I will explain that in a bit.

Many people assume that by drinking any fluid, they're ingesting water. While this is true to a certain extent, it is inherently deceiving. Many of the manufactured fluids such as soft drinks, energy drinks, and even some "juice drinks." (I say *juice drinks*, because they typically only contain 8-10% juice as well as chemicals instead of 100% juice.) They often consist of high amounts of sodium as well. While there may be H2O in these drinks, the sodium content creates a reverse effect and actually depletes your body of water.

Look at these labels from popular fruit drinks that contain less than twenty percent juice and a long list of chemicals (notice the sodium content of these items!):

Is it wrong to drink these types of drinks?

I will not tell you to completely quit enjoying a favored beverage, but it's a good place to start. According to the American Pediatrics Association, high calorie foods – in particular sodas and high calorie juices – are the leading cause of childhood and adult obesity.

So, how much water should you drink daily?

An outdated rule of thumb was called the "8 by 8" recommendation. The rule suggested that everyone drink 8 eight ounces of water per day. But the rule has proven to be flawed, since 8 by 8 is insufficient for most people and only applies to someone who lives a sedentary lifestyle. And since we are all about exercise and remaining physically and mentally active, the 8 by 8 rule does not apply here. **So, if you've heard it, forget it!**

Looking at this from a common sense perspective, we need to consider our intake of fluids as an investment in our overall health. Are beverages that contain outrageous amounts of calories, sugars, and high fructose corn syrup really worth it? These items are addictive and are designed to create *sensory reliance* – a craving for sweetness and familiar tastiness and the sugar rush they provide.

Another way to boost hydration is to eat vegetables with every meal which are high in water content and limited amounts of fruit, because of the sugar content. Fruits and vegetables, plus regular intake of water, will provide you with all the life-giving H2O your body constantly craves.

I suggest that when you wake up in the morning immediately drink a full glass of water. By doing so, you are replenishing up to 60% of your cells' needs. Trust me, you'll feel better as you start your day, you will find that your mind will be miraculously sharper and more clear, and long term you will be protecting yourself from illnesses that have been linked to chronic dehydration:

- High blood pressure
- Kidney and bladder infections
- Coronary heart disease
- High cholesterol
- Colon cancer
- Weight gain
- Obesity

I therefore also recommend that, before <u>every</u> meal, you drink a full 8 ounce glass of water. The water speeds your metabolism and aids swift digestion. In addition, you're playing a "trick" on your brain since receptors in your stomach will send a message to it that your stomach is "full." Consider water your inexpensive, healthful gastric bypass!

This is one of the simplest weight loss techniques but you normally will not hear this trick from weight-loss gurus. After all, water does not sell their programs.

To summarize, water is life. We need water to function no matter what, where, or how we do anything. It is imperative that we consume copious amounts of water on a daily basis.

My suggestion for you today is to start measuring your water intake. Just carry a simple pad and pen and every time you drink water, document it. At the end of the day, add up the water you drank. You may also want to keep notes on the fresh vegetables and fruits you eat.

Remember, every time we sweat and urinate, we lose water. But we also lose water when we are in stress. Just by relaxing, and eliminating the hate and negative elements around you and breathing can help your body keep its hydration levels at normal levels.

Remember this fact: if you are feeling thirst, you are already dehydrated. Do not allow yourself to feel thirst. Keep water with you at all times no matter where you are. Do not fool yourself into believing that humidity is keeping you hydrated. The rain or snow does not keep the body hydrated (snow and cold actually dehydrate bodies faster than the heat).

RULE OF THUMB: a bottle of water should be as much of a must-have as your smartphone. You should never have one without the other, preferably with the water bottle in your hand wherever you go.

CHAPTER SIX

*"Be miserable. Or motivate yourself. Whatever has to be done,
it's always your choice."*
-Wayne Dyer, Motivational Speaker

The Granite Method– STEP THREE

Alas, now you can use your "finishing tool!"

So far, you've learned the importance of finding your Cause and hopefully you've started to narrow down a Cause that will drive you to Be It and in that way make great and positive changes in your life.

You've also learned about *The Granite Method* and how you should start building a plan for using your mallet to break away the stone holding you back from an active, attractive life. You should have started already getting to the core person you are inside and the person you want to be. My videos are designed to give you techniques you can use to identify your plan and start taking action. If you haven't taken the time to watch them, I highly recommend you make the time! Now!

In this book, we have also discussed how you can use your sculpting tool to make changes that will greatly improve your health through nutrition and hydration. Again, watch those videos!

Now, I will tell you about how to use your <u>finishing tool</u> to make improvements in your psyche that will support you in your quest to BE YOUR CAUSE. Again, I promise, there's no hocus-pocus, no brainwashing, no ridiculous philosophies you have to study, and no mumbo-jumbo languages you have to learn. This next section is from the heart and derived from my many years counseling clients on how to achieve radical, positive change. I call it being *Tara-fied*. I view it as the direct opposite of being terrified. Instead of scared of change, you'll embrace it. Instead of being disappointed at every turn, you'll find strength in the challenges you'll inevitably uncover.

Okay, are you ready? Prepare to be Tara-fied!

"Tara-fying" Overview

When I have described my concept of BE CAUSE to clients and audiences, the question I sometimes get is, "Don't you just mean WHY?" That question gets my most energetic, "NO!"

Why is merely the answer to a question, typically a narrow question.

"Why must I lose weight?"

"Why do I have to stop drinking soda?"

"Why do I want to be successful?"

Be Cause goes must deeper. Your Cause is not only a way of being now – that supplies all the answers to your *why* questions – it's also your life mission. Your reason for *being*.

The thing to keep in mind here is that your Cause is NOT EASY. Many of the steps are tough. Clearing away the granite is hard work and using your sculpting and finishing tools is precise and painstaking.

The Granite Method is not at all like all the *Seven Days To A Better Body* or *Make Millions Selling Condemned Houses* books. For one compelling reason: The Granite Method actually works, IF you work at it.

"Tara-fying" Explained

The simple way to imagine Tara-fying your life is by thinking of it as your life GPS. When you wake up in the morning, the first question you should ask yourself is:

- **Where am I going today?**
Am I making multiple stops? Is the journey I'm on going to take me where I want to go? Will this trip be scenic or through rough neighborhoods? Does it answer today's *why* questions? Will I have a positive impact on my life and the lives of people who are on the journey with me? You should view your destination as THE LIFE THAT AWAITS YOU!

- **Who am I taking with me?**
Will the people I'm traveling with/working with/dining

with be a POSITIVE influence on my day and my
Cause?

- **Is my vehicle (my body) properly
fueled and maintained?**

What will it take to make sure my vehicle is in prime
working order? Is it properly fueled? Is there water in the
radiator?

- **Embark on today's journey.**

You can expect your trip will be slowed or changed by
unpredictable or predictable obstacles. In those moments,
you can decide to scream at the obstruction, or turn
around and give up the journey, OR you can decide to
Tara-fy. If you're finding your desire to continue is
being challenged, focus on the destination and its place
in your Cause. Use visualization to focus on positives,
like looking at the surroundings or playing music, to
bring you to a positive place. Use your companions
(those strictly positive ones you picked before you left!)
to distract you and support you.

You should trust that driving will be hard on you. But
you must push through, relying on the fact that you've
been working to make it easier and that the journey gets
easier over time.

When those negative thoughts creep in, identify them as
being negative and EXTERNAL to you, THAT
THEY'RE AN ILLUSION, and refuse to believe them!
Speak to them and say things like:

"Nice try! But you're not winning!"

"I choose to go in the right direction!"

"I AM BETTER THAN THAT!"

Should you fail and can't fight the negatives, you should hold yourself accountable but don't give in! It is NOT a pattern and it does NOT define you. YOU MUST PROMISE TO YOURSELF to try the journey again and again until it is second nature.

Also look at these moments as an opportunity to build self-confidence and self-esteem. The more you don't give up, the tougher you'll get, road warrior!

Be confident that the more you embark on these journeys, the negatives will visit you less and less because they will not have a chance to divert you. The obstacles will be fewer and you will look forward to that moment in the morning when you're setting your GPS to take you farther, to more luxurious destinations.

Leaving the road warrior metaphor, the concept applies to everything and anything that's part of your short-term goals and your Cause.

Sam from Nevada had spent so much of his time during his first week at the new technology company doing things that did not move him down the road. He spent hours organizing the office's accounting records, he became the lunch room's best joke teller. But nothing got him closer to his Cause: making money to support his family. It was only when he transformed himself from the Joker to one of the Aces in his company's metaphorical deck of cards that he moved closer to his destination. Sam eventually became the firm's most valuable cold-caller **when he finally picked up his hundred-pound cell phone.** Once he faced his fear, imagined his destination, and Tarafied his way of thinking.

*

The central messages from the Tara-fy concept are that fear and failure are illusions. You are worth a better life. You can make the changes you seek. You can live your Cause and you can love all the journeys to get you there.

The other message is: you are not alone. I will always be here. Because when you don't believe in yourself, I will always believe in you. You can trust that.

CHAPTER SEVEN

*"Think in the morning. Act in the noon. Eat in the
evening. Sleep in the night."*
-William Blake, Poet

It's as essential as water and, like with water, many of us
are desperately deficient of it.

Sleep.

The lack of it can steal our creative and intellectual
abilities, the serious lack of it will drive us mad and can
even kill us, either indirectly by causing illness and
disease or directly by causing our bodies to shut down.

The many tasks and responsibilities in our lives seem to
force us too often, though, to stay awake late into the
night or wake up long before our family and friends do,
and even medicate ourselves with caffeine and
amphetamines or cocaine so we can "power through." I
have heard some people say that sleep is overrated, and
that we should be able to function on 2-3 hours of sleep.

 While I often wish I had more hours in the day, I know
from my own experience and from hearing from my
clients that sleep is NOT overrated. Sleep IS important.

Earlier in this book, I explained how our bodies are
finely tooled machines. Machinery cannot run 24 hours a
day, 7 days per week without having times of rest. Our

bodies also need rest... we must sleep.

Yes, it would be great if we did not have to sleep an average of 25 years of our life away, but without sleep, we would be useless to ourselves, our families, and our employers. Sleep replenishes many parts of our body that we depleted during a normal day.

According to the National Sleep Foundation, sleep is essential for each person's health and overall well being, but a majority of us do not get the sleep we need. Some of the sleep deprivation is from our free will – we chose to eek out as much time as we can from the day – but for others, the sleep deprivation comes from physical disorders. And, according to the American Psychological Association, there are over 70 different sleep disorders with many sufferers having never been diagnosed. Some of the primary sleep disorders are:

- Sleep Apnea
- Chronic Insomnia
- Jet-Lag Syndrome
- Restless Leg Syndrome
- Delayed sleep-wake phase disorder
- Obesity hypo-ventilation syndrome

Essentially, though, the main cause of the majority of sleep related issues reverts back to what I have talked about throughout this book... balancing our lifestyles.

If we understand our Cause, we will have less stress in knowing where we are traveling to in life's journey and the steps we need to take to get there. This alone can help us sleep better.

Cutting down on the decisions we need to make in a day, a week, or a month's time can also help our sleep activity. If we are always thinking about the next decision, we are creating an unneeded stress that can cause an imbalance of sleep. We may think we are sleeping, but when our mind is overloaded with choices, we are not getting the healthy REM sleep our minds and bodies need for survival.

I mentioned looking inside and reaching outside, and if you are suffering from sleep deprivation, this could be the time you need to speak with a sleep professional. There is nothing wrong with seeking counsel for an issue that is affecting your life. I suggest telling your family doctor, and I am sure he/she can suggest either a sleep counselor or specialist, or possibly a psychologist. Allowing a sleep issue to go too long without treatment can lead to very serious mental and physical problems.

I spoke about the basic laws of the body, and sleep is one of those basic laws. A human cannot go without proper sleep and keep their sanity. Sometimes the best way to attain good sleep is to adjust our diets. There are foods and liquids that can challenge the healthy sleep we need. One of the largest culprits of this is caffeine. Many sleep professionals have solved patient's sleep issues just by cutting down their caffeine intake. A large amount of those individuals would state they do not drink coffee, thinking it was the only caffeine-laden item. Caffeine is in many of the foods and drinks that we ingest daily. Knowing what items have caffeine is a good first step in recognizing how to change your diet for healthier sleep patterns. And, the FDA does not require manufacturers to state how much caffeine is in products. Here are some surprising sources of caffeine:

- **Decaffeinated coffee is not completely free of caffeine.** Tests have shown it does have less than normal coffee, but it is not completely free of the substance.
- **Chocolate is a prime source of caffeine.** It is naturally within our favorite chocolate bars.
- **Many weight loss pills use caffeine** as the primary ingredient to cut hunger.
- **Pain relief medication** is another source of high levels of caffeine. If you are taking over-the-counter medicine for migraine headaches, there is a good chance it has caffeine.
- **Energy drinks and energy water** is another source of high caffeine. Not all brands use caffeine, but a large percentage create the "energy" via caffeine.

Some individuals have even thought they could replace their coffee with tea. The majority of teas have more caffeine than coffee.

Any item on store shelves that states it can create energy should be suspected of containing caffeine. If you read the ingredients carefully, you will probably discover I am correct.

Sleep studies have shown that we deplete some key resources in our brains and that the only way these resources are repaired and replenished is with sleep. If a person does not get a proper night's sleep, they are actually better off choosing to sleep over choosing to exercise, because if the brain is not repaired, the body will not react to the exercise.

Additionally, it is during the last stage of our sleep cycle when a secretion of hormones occurs. This secretion controls a large part of our metabolism, and actually performs a physical repair of our bodies. When we miss out on this sleep, our bodies are not receiving the maintenance and repair they need.

The stages of sleep are:

•   **Stage 1:** You have your eyes closed and are in an easy position to be awakened. This should last on average, 5 to 10 minutes.
•   **Stage 2:** You have entered a light sleep pattern where your heart rate begins to slow down and your body temperature drops. You are preparing for deep sleep.
•   **Stage 3:** This is the most critical stage when you have entered a deep sleep stage. The body is being repaired by the secretion of hormones, and if awakened, this causes a "malfunction" in the repair and maintenance functions our minds and bodies were developed with.

REM sleep usually happens at different periods during the sleep stages. Normally, the first REM occurrence happens approximately 90 minutes after falling asleep. It is during REM sleep that dreams occur. If you are an individual who believes you do not have dreams, it could mean you are not sleeping well and not entering the REM stages.

Studies have also shown that many cases of depression are due to the lack of REM (Rapid Eye Movement) sleep. During REM sleep, your eyes move very fast back and forth and your brain is actually both exercising and repairing major components of your body. The resulting depression from a serious lack of REM can lead to overeating and less frequent physical activities.

So yes, sleep is very important to our overall well being... mind, body, emotions, mood, overall well-being. If we are not sleeping properly, our minds and bodies will not react the way they were designed to.

Just like our daily work and play activities for which we set schedules, we need to do the same with our sleep. If we go to sleep at irregular times, we confuse our bodies and minds. While it is sometimes difficult keeping schedules, it is healthy to set a sleep schedule, going to bed at the same time every night, and optimally to wake up at the same time.

So what is more important, quality or quantity of sleep? Both are important, but quality is probably taking a slight lead. The average adult should get 7 to 8 hours of sleep daily, but if their sleep environment is optimal (noise and interruption free), 6 hours may be sufficient. The key is a high quality in which the person enters all stages of sleep and is easily detected since he or she should waken feeling satisfied with being awake. If you feel a desire to keep sleeping every time you awaken, you just might not be getting the quality sleep your body needs.

Watch my videos for this chapter on the little and big things you can do to make sure the quality and quantity of your sleep are the best they can be. Look for my videos about natural sleep-inducing substances like ginger root and melatonin that can work wonders!

 So to reiterate, sleep is as important, or even more important than daily exercise. You can run, walk, do push-ups and pull-ups day in and day out, but if you are not getting proper and healthy sleep, you are nullifying all the exercise!

A MILLION POUNDS IN MISSISSIPPI

"I've struggled with my weight for years. Having Tara as a health coach and mentor has been a huge blessing in my life."
-Ronald Evans

"Tara is SO supportive. She keeps me motivated and on target."
-Bernard Jordan

"To date, I have lost nearly 20 pounds, within about a one month time frame, and I feel better than I've felt in a long time."
-Rosa Jordan

So why Mississippi? After all, I am from New Jersey, but there is an inner call that told me to start with what is considered the State with the highest rate of obesity.

There are many issues in the world and in the United States in this era, but the one problem that I believe needs to be a priority is the health and well-being of the human population. After all, how can any of us fix other issues if we are not healthy enough to do so?

My goal is to see 1,000,000 pounds leave Mississippi, and it has started. The pounds are leaving.

Many may ask, why is obesity such a problem in

Mississippi? I have news for you, obesity is a problem nationwide. In the 1980's, obesity levels were sitting at 15% or lower in each and every State. Now, there are no States lower than a 21% obesity level, and well over 10 States are over the 30% mark.

When I look at the obesity levels in Mississippi, I can somewhat understand. When I enter this wonderful Southern State, I can smell the odors of great cooking. And, Mississippians do like to eat. Don't we all?

But exercise does not seem to be high on the agenda. The State scores low on daily activity and when we eat and sit, the pounds just stay on us.

Mississippi is also the poorest State in the nation. This can also lead to people eating calorie-filled foods instead of healthy fruits and vegetables. This is because the high calorie food items seem to be cheaper at the supermarkets. Therefore, we have people eating foods high in cholesterol, carbohydrates and other items that create obesity, and not eating foods high in vitamins and minerals that can lead to good health.

As I was moved to tears for some of my fellow human beings, I looked even deeper into the health problems in the State of Mississippi.

And, I found no surprises. There are high rates of diseases like diabetes and heart disease. Hyper-tension is a major issue.

I asked myself why? Why are the residents of Mississippi treating their bodies this way? Why are they shortening their life spans? And the answer was right in front of me. It is an answer that is evident for many of the problems in the world...it is what we know. It is the way we were raised and we know no different way.

The inner voice came.

"Tara, you need to go show them a different way."

I am a person that listens when that inner voice speaks, so with a goal of seeing 1,000,000 unwanted Mississippi pounds disappear, I traveled to the State of Mississippi.

And, I was welcomed with open arms and smiles. I met many people who know that their health is important, they just needed a teacher...a mentor...a friend.

Well, let me tell you, we are watching Mississippi pounds being eradicated quickly and safely.

My Mississippi friends are still eating great recipes, but they are adding the fruits and vegetables that are needed. They are following strict, and fun exercise schedules. And I am seeing depression being turned into smiles.

But, Mississippi is not the only State that is confronting the obesity epidemic. All throughout the Southern States, we discover higher rates of obesity. Some blame this trend on the culture...eating fried chicken, fried green tomatoes, fried pickles, and many other fried things. But this can turn into a system of putting groups of people all in one box. It can be discriminatory and when we assume the obesity is just tied to the culture, we will bypass many individuals who are having weight problems for other reasons.

There are obese people in every State and country in the world, and we need to look at individual circumstances each time. What may help one person may not help the next. But there are certain steps we can all take to start the process, and I aim to share them on my blog and by traveling to various locations to show people healthier alternatives.

While diets are a major contributor to obesity, lack of physical activity comes in at a close second. In some cases, individuals need to be shown some ways to exercise and use their bodies without being forced to pay large amounts of money to do so. Just simply walking instead of driving can be a good example. Or, working a garden in which you are using physical abilities to grow healthy items for you and your family's diets.

I will state that I am seeing improvements in thought patterns about obesity, but we all need to make a concerted effort to show and help each other in the obesity epidemic. Not only in Mississippi, but in the complete nation.

We have reasons to be optimistic. I have watched many of my new-found friends in Mississippi losing pounds in healthy ways. I have a goal of spreading this across the nation.

Mississippi is State #1 and 49 States to go. If 1,000,000 pounds can be swept away in Mississippi, it makes sense that we can erase 50,000,000 pounds in the United States. And have fun doing so!

CONCLUSION

*"I believe that the greatest gift you can give your family
and the world
is a healthy you."*
-Joyce Mayer, Motivational Author

So here we are. At the end of this book. I'll more
correctly call it, though, the beginning.

I have introduced you to a few things between these
pages, most notably being the urgent task ahead of you –
to find, if you haven't already done so, your awe-
inspiring, obstacle-shattering, results-driven CAUSE and
ways for you to BE IT.

I've provided you with some incentives to take action to
improve your physical and mental states, and in my
videos I've been giving you specific tips, information,
and inspirations to get moving! Trust me, I won't think
less of you if you started small. There is nothing
shameful about that. There is only shame in doing
nothing at all.

*"If you dream of something worth doing and then
simply go to work on it and don't think anything of
personalities, or emotional conflicts, or of money,
or of family distractions; it is amazing how quickly you
get
through those 5,000 steps."*
-Edwin Land, Inventor of the Polaroid Camera

I am looking forward to getting to know all of you. I am committed to answering your questions and meeting you someday. Be sure to take BEFORE pictures! And you can share them with me, if you like. (I promise never to post or share anything without your permission!) I am committed to each and every one of you – my heart is set on seeing your progress first hand and helping you through every challenge.

You can do it! I know you can.

Just like Candice did!

"How do I look?" Candice said to me the first time I saw her after she'd taken a trip around the world.

Candice, after having lost two hundred fifteen pounds *being her cause*, decided she needed to show off her new body and an amazing outlook on life that had emerged after she made radical changes to her body and her mental state. Candice took a "Victory Tour," as she called it – a river cruise up and down the rivers flowing into the Mediterranean. She was gone nearly a month. I frequently received email updates from her, reporting of the many men she had met during the trip, and the occasional "summer loves" who were knocking on her newly polished granite statue.

"You look amazing, honey," I choked, tears flowing from my eyes.

Her sun-bleached hair matched her golden tan perfectly and her rosy cheeks were less about the sun and more about a happiness that shown now from within her.

"Did you find love, like you had hoped?" I asked.

"I did, Tara," she responded. "For the first time in my life, I love who I am."

Candice still stops in to see me, whenever she feels the need for inspiration or whenever I find myself overwhelmed keeping up with the research of the day. Candice can sense when I'm tempted to violate my own rules about sleep. She always brings me two bottles of water, slightly cooler than room temperature, and a small square of dark chocolate. After all, Candice knows the power of sweet rewards, always in moderation.

To think how far Candice has come, and how far <u>you</u> can go!

I leave you for now with a quote that always inspires me…

> **"Nothing is impossible, the word itself says 'I'm possible'!"**
> -Audrey Hepburn, Actress/ Philanthropist

Your vision for yourself is possible. Be your Cause. Take action. It only takes one step at a time.

With love and admiration,
Tara

ABOUT THE AUTHOR

Tara Christopher has been in the health and fitness industry for nearly thirty years. She started as a competitive AAU swimmer at the age of five, swimming five days a week, and completing her first swim-a-thon at age nine. She continues organizing swim-a-thons annually to raise money for various non-profit organizations.

At twelve years of age, Tara's participated in her first twenty-mile walk-a-thon, instilling in her a strong awareness of the importance of fitness and good health especially in the context of helping others.

Tara began teaching aerobics, and was part of a team that opened a health club at the age of seventeen. While opening the new health club, McDonald's was attempting to incorporate a veggie-burger into its menu; Tara was selected to be the spokesperson for the McDonalds commercial to help launch the concept of a healthier choice.

At age twenty-one, Tara competed in her first sprint triathlon and was featured on the cover of the Triathlon program as the cyclist.

After moving locations to teach weight training and aerobics classes, Tara was invited to speak at the corporate office of Anheuser Busch, to inspire a room full of upper management to educate them on exercise and better nutrition. This was the first of many engagements to teach health and wellness.

After receiving her bachelor's degree from Hunter College, Tara launched a successful career at an exclusive gym in an upscale neighborhood in New York City. Her mission was to develop programs for individuals to reach their goals based on their own health needs. Following rapid growth and success working with highly demanding clients, Tara launched her own business on in Manhattan at Lift gym = While in the process of launching her business, Tara finished the NYC marathon. Since then, she has completed many endurance events including the Ford Ironman.

Throughout her career, Tara has been featured in multiple national publications; she was in an exercise layout in Fitness Plus; she wrote a television clip for Life Time Live; she was featured in that episode; and she was chosen to represent the book Baby to Bikini, traveling to many news morning shows. In 2012, Tara was featured on Dateline NBC as "The Coach". After the showing, the clip was featured on TMZ and the O'Reilly factor.

With social media and the changing formats for how to reach global audiences, Tara has been inspired to reach out to people with her message. In various business settings, Tara has distinguished herself as a leader, having been given multiple awards for exemplary professional achievement. In 2016, she was nominated for an outstanding woman in business by the Leading Women Entrepreneurs and Business Owners organization.

This has led to her passion to spread the word in her first book, *50 Million Pounds In America*.